Intermittent fasting

Guide For Women Over 50

2 Books In 1

Learn To Lose Weight, Detox Your Body, Increase Longevity And Improve Well-Being With The Method That's Right For You (16:8, 5:2, 12:12).

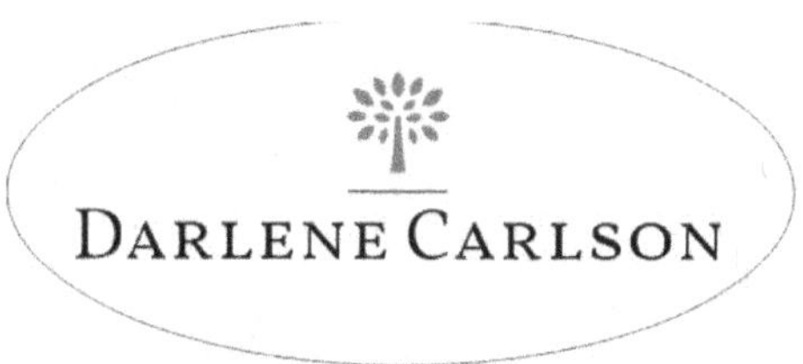

DARLENE CARLSON

Thank you for purchasing the book,

After reading it, I would be grateful if you could take a minute of your time to leave an honest Amazon review about my work and share your experience with other customers.

Thank you!

Table of Contents

INTRODUCTION

Fad diets thrive in the world. Diet pills were common in the 1990s. You were losing out on life's classic health supplements if you didn't have a juicer in the early 2000s. Green tea pads that lower tummy size have been given to us, and if you're not eating like a Neanderthal, you're still at a disadvantage. As a rule, I'm cynical of all fads. If something is marketed as ground-breaking in weight loss, it's probably just a marketing hack to sell whatever is popular at the time. If there was ever a fad to get on board with, it's intermittent fasting.

Intermittent fasting includes alternating between cycles of fasting and feeding, and it's become increasingly common in recent years. It was not only the "most common" weight loss google search in 2019, but it was also featured prominently in a review article published in The New England Journal of Medicine.

If performed correctly, intermittent fasting can have important health benefits, including losing the weight, type 2 diabetes recovery, and many other items. It can also help you save time and money.

Chapter 1
What Is Intermittent Fasting?

Intermittent fasting is the method of limiting calorie consumption by following a set of rules that includes both on and off feeding times. It can seem boring and easy at first, but once you give it a try, you can see the advantages of fasting in your everyday life. It is a self-discipline exercise that can be challenging in the beginning. Weight loss, mental stability, a good night's sleep, and a lot of energy have all been recorded by people who have tried intermittent fasting. Intermittent fasting has long been known to help people lose belly fat. Since it's difficult to see decreased fat areas on the body, the loss of belly fat is mostly due to hormones, and as we all know, weight storage in the mid-section is a part of life during menopause.

People who choose to remain younger use intermittent fasting for extended periods of time. Prof. David Sinclair of Harvard University, a longevity expert and scientist, made the following comment. "No one knows the exact solution or the ideal fasting process, even though they claim to." According to studies on mice, eating 30% less food increases lifespan by 30%. You will get stressed if you listen to all the experts and understand all of the nuances.

Intermittent fasting (IF) is a form of eating that alternates between fasting and regular eating. Fasting on alternating days, regular 16-hour fasts, or fasting for 24 hours two days a week are the most common approaches. Both intermittent fasting regimens will be referred to as intermittent fasting in this article. Intermittent fasting, unlike most diets, does not require calorie or macronutrient monitoring. There are no limits on what foods you can consume or avoid, because it's more like a way of life than a diet.

Intermittent fasting is a common way to lose weight because it is an easy, quick, and efficient way to eat very little and lose body fat.

It may also aid in the prevention of diabetes and heart disease, the maintenance of muscle mass, and the improvement of psychological well-being.

Furthermore, since there are less meals to schedule, prepare, and cook, this eating style will help you reduce time in the kitchen.

Intermittent fasting – isn't that starvation?

No, fasting varies from starving in one important way: it allows you to maintain control. The unintentional avoidance of food for an extended period of time is known as starvation. It can result in excruciating pain or even death. It's neither planned nor orchestrated. Fasting, on the other hand, is the voluntary abstention from eating for moral, nutritional, or other purposes. It's carried out by someone who isn't naturally thin and has enough accumulated body fat to last a lifetime. Fasting should never cause pain and should never result in death if performed correctly.

You have access to food, but you just choose to not consume it. It may be for any length of time, from a few hours to a few days, or even a week or more if medical supervision is provided. You can start whenever you want, and you can end it whenever you want.

Intermittent fasting is where you don't eat for a while. You might, for example, fast from dinner to breakfast, a span of 12-14 hours. Intermittent fasting must be considered a part of daily life in this way.

Look at the word "breakfast." It relates to the meal that you eat to break your fast, which you do every day. Rather than being a cruel and inhumane, the English language means that fasting should be undertaken on a daily basis, even though it is only for a brief amount of time.

Intermittent fasting isn't anything out of the ordinary; it's a way of life for several people. It is, without a doubt, the most ancient and successful dietary intervention ever invented. We have somehow underestimated its healing potential and lost its influence. Learning how to fast correctly helps one to choose whether or not to do it.

1.1 Intermittent Fasting for Weight Loss

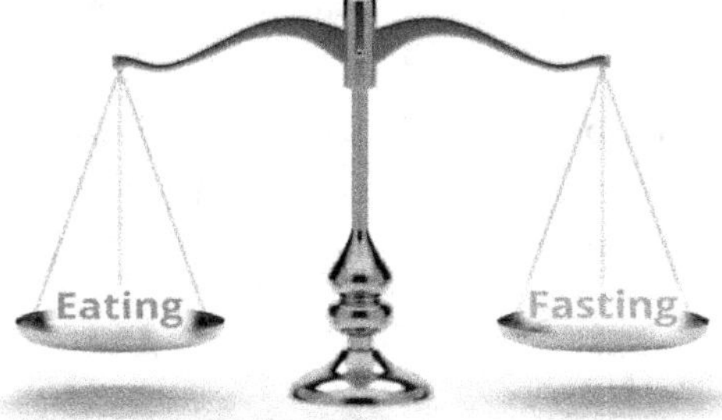

Intermittent fasting, at the simplest form, helps the body to use its surplus energy by consuming extra body fat.

It's important to note that this is natural, and humans have adapted to fast for shorter periods of time – hours or days – without having harmful health effects. Food energy has been accumulated in the form of body fat. Your body would actually "eat" the fat for energy if you don't eat. Life is all about finding the right balance. The yin and the yang, the positive and the negative. The same is so when it comes to fasting and eating. Overall, fasting is just the reverse of feeding. You are fasting if you are not fed.

When we consume, we use more nutritional calories than we can use right now. A part of this energy must be retained for later use. Insulin is a hormone that helps the body store energy from food.

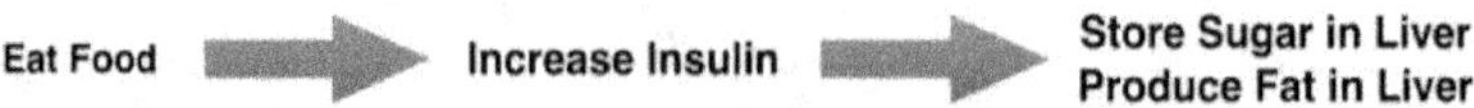

Insulin levels increase as we feed, assisting in the storage of surplus energy in two ways. Specific glucose (sugar) units are broken down and joined into long chains to form glycogen, which is contained in the liver or muscle.

However, there is a finite amount of storage capacity for sugars, and once the limit is reached, the liver continues to convert the extra glucose to fat. De novo lipogenesis is the name given to this process ("making new fat").

The liver retains some of the freshly produced fat, but the rest of it is distributed to other fatty tissue in the body. Although this is a more difficult operation, the amount of fat produced is almost limitless.

In our bodies, we have two important food energy storage mechanisms. One is easy to access but has minimal storage space (Glycogen), while the other is harder to access but has almost infinite storage space (body fat).

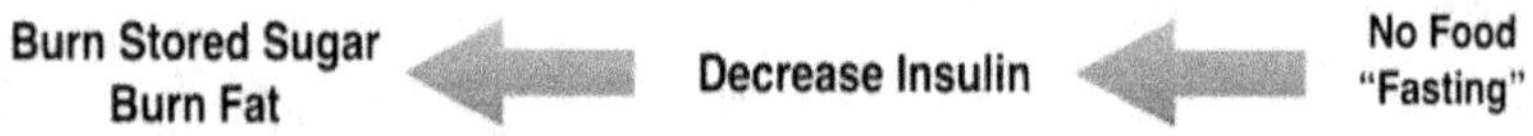

When we don't eat, the mechanism reverses. Insulin levels drop, signalling the body to begin consuming stored energy because food is no longer available. Since blood glucose levels are falling, the body should now draw glucose from storage to use for energy. Glycogen is the most readily available source of electricity.

To supply sugar to the body's other cells, it is broken down into glucose molecules. It has enough resources to satisfy much of the body's needs for 24 to 36 hours. After that, the body's primary source of nutrition would be fat breakdown. As a result, there are only two states in which the body will exist: fed and fasted. We are either processing food energy or wasting energy that has been stored (decreasing stores). It's either this or that. There must be no net weight difference if feeding and fasting are matched.

We waste nearly half of our life in the fed state if we start feeding as soon as we get out of bed and don't stop until we go to sleep. We may accumulate weight over time because we haven't given our bodies enough time to burn stored food fat.

We will only need to boost the amount of time we spend burning food energy to regain balance or lose weight. Intermittent fasting is what it's called.

Intermittent fasting, in turn, enables the body to use its remaining fat. What's important to remember is that there's nothing incorrect with that. That is the way our bodies are made. Dogs, lions, bears, and cats all do this. That's what people do.

Your body will constantly use the incoming food resources if you feed every third hour, which is frequently advised. It might not be appropriate to burn much, if any, body fat. It's likely that you're actually storing fat.

It's possible that your body is storing it until a moment when you won't be able to feed. If this occurs, you are out of control. You're losing out on intermittent fasting.

1.2 How Intermittent Fasting Helps You Lose Weight

There are some weight-loss advantages of eating this way. The first is that your body will be pushed to use accumulated body fat for energy while you're fasting. After a few hours without food, the body can deplete its sugar reserves, causing it to turn to burning fat for energy, a mechanism known as metabolic switching. Mark Mattson, Ph.D., a Johns Hopkins neuroscientist, describes the result in basic terms: "Intermittent fasting varies from the usual feeding routine of most Americans, who feed constantly during the day... When anyone consumes three meals a day, plus snacks, and does not exercise, they are storing calories rather than burning fat reserves every time they feed."

Caloric expenditure this way, rather than from the meals you consume during the day, can aid in substantial weight loss, as well as weight loss from any extra body fat you may have.

It says you'll not only be lighter, but you'll still look and feel better than you would if you lost weight the traditional way.

Intermittent fasting will help you get the best out of your body's fat-burning hormones. Human growth hormone (HGH) and insulin are two of the most essential hormones.

Human growth hormone is essential for switching on your body's fat-burning furnace so that it can get the calories it needs from stored body fat to function and play. Fasting has been shown in studies to boost HGH productivity dramatically.

The impact of intermittent fasting on insulin is equally as impressive, if not more so. It's crucial to keep your insulin levels down and stable if you want to lose weight to keep it off. Processed carbohydrate (bread, pasta, rice) and basic sugar (cookies, sweets, and soda)-rich diets have the opposite effect. Any time you consume one of these things, your insulin levels increase quickly and then crash. As a result of this phenomenon, the body can retain more of what you consume as excess body fat rather than burning it as energy. Elevating the insulin levels in this way for a long time will lead to type 2 diabetes, obesity, and other chronic health issues. Intermittent fasting is an easy solution to this problem.

Men who fasted intermittently had "dramatically lower insulin levels and greatly increased insulin sensitivity," according to one report.

Since you haven't given your body enough food, it won't release insulin, causing insulin levels to stabilize before you eat again. It keeps the body in a fat and calorie-burning mode. It will also provide you with more energy during the day.

Another great weight losing advantage of fasting is that appetite pangs and cravings would be reduced, if not completely gone. Its ability to regulate the insulin and blood sugar levels, as well as to fix other hormonal imbalances, is most likely the cause. How Does Intermittent Fasting Help Weight Loss?

1.3 WOMEN AND FASTING

Are women capable of fasting? Or is it – like many people already say – potentially detrimental to them?

Fasting for losing weight has a long tradition, which is unsurprising. It is understandable that if you do not eat, you will lose weight.

Which makes people's fear of skipping even a single meal, let alone fasting for a day or more, all the more shocking. Some people worry that fasting will cause them to go into hunger mode and gain weight. That's akin to claiming that splashing water on your head would make your hair dry. It's a bit of a Bizarro universe. It's a lie used to frighten people.

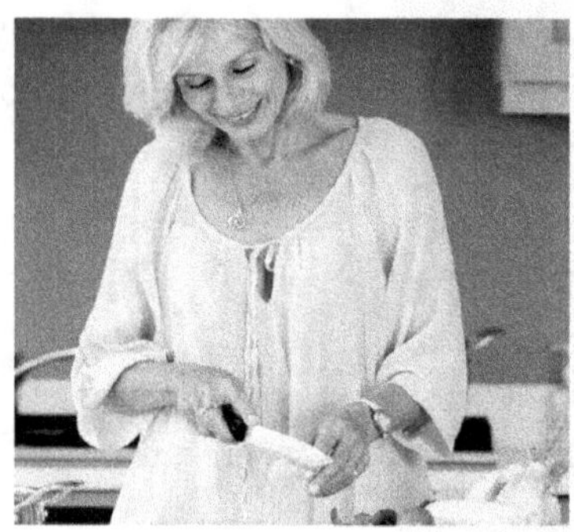

There are several accounts of people's metabolisms being ruined. Of necessity, food marketers have enthusiastically 'trained' medical experts explaining the risks of skipping meals and the benefits of sugar consumption. When you miss meals, no one makes money.

A Long History of Fasting

Fasting was first recorded in medical literature over a century ago. It cites 'trained fasters,' who can fast for particular times for exhibition purposes. One practitioner went on a 30-day fast and drank his own urine. What a case of being bored out of your mind. It's a bit like watching time pass. In Franz Kafka's fantasy novel "A Hunger Artist," it is represented.

From 1883 to 1924, fasting for entertainment was popular. Drs. Folin and Denis defined fasting as a "clean, healthy, and useful strategy for losing the weight of those who are obese" in the early 1900s. This is awesome. That is precisely what we need. Anything that is both secure and reliable.

Fasting has been done for thousands of years (mostly for religious reasons), which only contributed to the long tradition of protection. Fasting has been practiced for 5,000 years, so it's difficult to say that it's unhealthy. It's also plausible to argue that using soap is bad. Despite this, there are many misconceptions regarding the hazards of fasting.

Dr. W. Bloom reinvigorated interest in fasting as a preventive measure in the early 1950s, but with shortened fasting times. However, the literature still mentions several longer stretches.

FASTING FOR WOMEN?

Dr. Gilliland discussed the resurgence of fasting in the 1950s and 1960s, and his encounter with 46 patients "for whom the decreasing regime began with a regular absolute fast for 14 days." People's eyes nearly pop out of their heads when it's mentioned that they fast for even more than 24 hours; these people had 'standard' fast that stretched two weeks! And that was just the start. There were 14 men and 32 women among them.

It's vital to consider if fasting works for women. It's mainly because of an online article that's been seen over 100,000 times. This is what she wrote in 2012 – "Women and intermittent fasting: Can women fast? The few experiments that have been performed indicate that the answer is no." This could not be further from the facts. Hundreds of researches covering over 100 years, as well as professional practice spanning 5,000 years, indicate that women and men react similarly, with the exception of being underweight.

It's a simple problem. Is it appropriate for someone who is significantly underweight to fast? No way. That doesn't need you to be a genius to find out. Yes, you will become infertile if you are undernourished or underweight and fast.

Take a look back at the last 2,000 years of civilization. Is it true that Muslim women are excluded from fasting? Is it true that Buddhist women are excluded from fasting? Is it correct that Catholic women are excluded from fasting? No, it's not real. As a result, we have millions of people-years of experience working with women and fasting. And in 99.9% of the cases, there are no concerns.

There is no substantial disparity between males and females in a clinic where the doctor treated up to 1,000 people. Women, on the whole, do well. It seems that men are often just huge infants. The highest success rates have been found as husband and wife work together.

Exceptions and problems

In virtually all human religions, however, pregnant women and their children are 'free' from fasting. This is absolutely rational in all cases. Human cultures have already accepted that these individuals have higher growth needs.

Let's be explicit about something. Fasting in women causes a number of issues, according to this point. They do, however, produce men, and they do so quickly. Women don't necessarily lose weight the manner they want. Men, too, are subject to this. Amenorrhea is a condition that occurs when fat is too poor. That isn't a dilemma that we can solve by fasting.

If you have amenorrhea or really any symptoms when fasting, stop immediately. This is your body's way of reminding you that you require additional nutrients. Then there's the issue of eating disorders. It is more common in women due to the misconception that they are most likely to experience from eating disorders. Who, though, is not gender-specific? Do not fast if you have an eating disorder. It doesn't matter who you are.

In the first fourteen days, the patients were admitted to a metabolic ward and given only water, tea, and coffee. They were then released and told to stick to 600-1,000 calories daily.

Surprisingly, two patients demanded to be allowed to return for a second 14-day fasting cycle because they expected improved outcomes. Was it successful? Is there any way to tell if there was ever any doubt?

In 14 days, the total weight loss was 17.2 lbs. (8 kg). Fasting over extended periods of time results in weight reduction of around 1/2 pound (0.2 kg) per day. It implies that some of the original weight loss is due to water loss. The fast weight gain after refeeding confirms this hypothesis.

It's vital to realize this in order to stop the discomfort that always comes with weight gain when you eat again. The rapid weight loss and gain is water weight, not a sign that the fasting was unsuccessful. The 2-week fasting cycle was fulfilled by 44 of the 46 patients. One became nauseous, and the other chose not to continue and bowed out. And with a two-week fasting routine, that's a 96 percent success rate! It is also our professional practice. People still believe they can't do it despite never having attempted it. Patients in our Comprehensive Dietary Management (IDM) program soon learn that fasting is simple once we get started. Patients were advised to eat a low-calorie diet after the fasting time was over. It didn't work out. During the two-year follow-up phase, half of the patients did not stick to the diet. Instead of using the efficient sporadic methods we addressed in the previous article, they went back to the inadequate continuous energy constraint.

The important thing to remember is that life's normal rhythm is Feast and Fast. There are occasions when you should eat (weddings, ceremonies) and times when you should fast (holidays). It comes and goes. Constantly restricting calories for years on end is unhealthy and, most importantly, ineffective.

Drenick1Ketones first emerged in the urine on day two and stayed in the urine for the remainder of the fast. By the end of the two weeks, all three diabetics were free of insulin. At the conclusion of the study, one patient with serious congestive heart problems was free to walk without gasping for air. This two-week fast was not only not dangerous, but also incredibly helpful, as we were advised.

Was it difficult? A 'feeling of wellness' and 'euphoria,' according to Dr. Gilliland. Are you hungry? No, no, and no "For the first day, there were no complaints of hunger. We didn't come into anorexia." Some scholars at the time shared these sentiments.

Dr. Drenick of the Los Angeles VA Medical Centre has also published widely about clinical fasting. In 1968, he wrote about his experiences. It was a time when people were rekindling their curiosity in fasting for weight loss. He wrote about his experiences with six men and four women. Was it successful? Yes, in a nutshell.

Is it appropriate for women to fast? Yes, really.

1.4 Tips for Getting Started

It's not easy to adjust to intermittent fasting, particularly if you're doing it all at once. During our feeding times, we must avoid overeating vast quantities of processed foods. We would not see any effects if we do this. It is suggested that you start by changing your eating habits. Before undertaking extended fasting, settling into a habit of eating as healthily as practicable would be incredibly helpful. Begin this two-week prior you decide to start your intermittent fasting routine, and it will make the transition even smoother. Staying concentrated can be tough, but here are few tips to help you keep on track. At night, you should avoid snacking. It is perhaps the most difficult task, and it is where I expended the majority of my resources. Feeling hunger throughout the day, on the other hand, is a reflection of the good you're doing to your body, as David Sinclair said it.

As a result, you should prepare your mind to embrace the slight hunger pangs during the day. Thinking and believing like it is for the better good of the human body is one way to go about it.

Himalayan rock salt will deceive the body into thinking it is not hungry. When you're hungry, take a couple of granules and stick them under your tongue to make you feel better.

Do not take any supplements when fasting as the body must be left to its own devices to do all the job.

When breaking a fast, the body responds by consuming protein. It does aid in compensating for calorie or energy loss.

If you have a busy day ahead of you, try doing a 20/4 fast so you don't have to think about food, meal preparation, or preparing. Depending on your schedule, you should switch fasting times. It's rewarding to hit the target. When you see the benefits of fasting, you'll want to do it again.

21 Day Intermittent Fasting CHALLENGE

Day 1	Day 2	Day 3	Day 4	Day 5	Day 6	Day 7
16h FAST / 8h EAT	16h FAST / 8h EAT	16h FAST / 8h EAT	16h FAST / 8h EAT	16h FAST / 8h EAT	16h FAST / 8h EAT	16h FAST / 8h EAT
MAKE A PROTEIN SMOOTHIE	HIGH PROTEIN LUNCH	JOIN 21 DAY HERO FB GROUP	GO FOR A WALK	DRINK BLACK COFFEE WHEN HUNGRY	HAVE TWO BIG MEALS	MAKE A NICE DINNER

Day 8	Day 9	Day 10	Day 11	Day 12	Day 13	Day 14
16h FAST / 8h EAT	16h FAST / 8h EAT	16h FAST / 8h EAT	18h FAST / 6h EAT	16h FAST / 8h EAT	16h FAST / 8h EAT	16h FAST / 8h EAT
REFLECT ON YOUR PROGRESS	EXERCISE FASTED	ADD GREENS TO PROTEIN SMOOTHIE	EXTEND YOUR FAST BY 2H	TRY BULLETPROOF COFFEE	SKIP SUGAR	MAKE A NICE DINNER

Day 15	Day 16	Day 17	Day 18	Day 19	Day 20	Day 21
16h FAST / 8h EAT	16h FAST / 8h EAT	16h FAST / 8h EAT	18h FAST / 8h EAT	16h FAST / 8h EAT	16h FAST / 8h EAT	18h FAST / 6h EAT
HIGH FIBER LUNCH	FULL BODY TRAINING	EAT ONLY WHOLE FOODS	EXERCISE FASTED	SKIP SUGAR	REFLECT ON YOUR PROGRESS	EXTEND YOUR FAST BY 2H

We developed a 21-Day Intermittent Fasting Plan to help you get started on your Fasting journey in a simple, enjoyable, and healthy manner. It provides action items for each day, as well as detailed overview and additional learnings.

Scroll down to get a sneak look at the first seven days of Intermittent Fasting. Join 21-day Intermittent Fasting Challenge if you believe it's time to take things within your own hand to make Intermittent Fasting a healthier approach. It provides you access to the whole 21-day Intermittent Fasting schedule, and additional Intermittent Fasting Beginner (and Advanced!) tips and tricks.

DAY 1

Task: 12h eat | 12h fast

Mission: Start the plan

You can gradually ease into intermittent fasting over the first week. This is why we recommend beginning with Twelve hours of fasting on Day 1 and gradually to 16 hours on Day 5 by introducing one hour of fasting per day. It would be better for the brain and body to adjust to the new food habits this way. You also allow yourself sufficient time to become accustomed to Intermittent Fasting.

You should pick the Intermittent Fasting plan that best suits your lifestyle and that you will observe for the whole 21-day Intermittent Fasting Challenge on the first day. Consistency has been found to be one of the most significant aspects in achieving success.

DAY 2

Task: 11h Eat | 13h Fast

Mission: Grip the basics

Your fast will be extended to 13 hours on Day 2. You should do it in just one hour more than you did yesterday!

Day 2 is a perfect day to start learning about balanced eating tips that will help you meet your Fasting goals: consume rich foods and skip the usual suspects like starch, refined foods, and empty carbohydrates.

It will give you a rundown of popular meals and foods that you should consume to improve your Intermittent Fasting outcomes. Consider simple, tasty, and well-balanced home-cooked meals like feta cheese salad, meatballs with zucchini noodles, poached eggs with spinach, or homemade hummus for a snack.

DAY 3

Task: 10h eat | 14h fast

Mission: Create the Rewards

When it comes to developing a new Intermittent Fasting habit, rewards are important. As a result, on Day 3, you would be able to choose your incentives for each successfully fasted day. What is the significance of rewards? A reward sends a message to the brain that says, "It feels nice to be doing this. It's what we can do more of! ".. Everything which makes you happy then do it.

Intermittent Fasting rewards should ideally be linked to your primal needs for relaxation, social interaction, sleep, or play.

Alternatively, the reward may be a quick (but powerful!) celebratory gesture you take right after finishing the habit, such as patting yourself on the back and saying "Good work," or crossing another day off the everyday progress report form.

If the incentive is more substantial, such as a lunch at an expensive yet delectable restaurant, you can use the token strategy, in which each good day of fasting "gives you" one token. You should treat yourself to a meal at the restaurant.

DAY 4

Task: 9h Eat | 15h Fast

Mission: Take a protein lunch

On Day 4 of Fasting, you'll already have fasted for 15 hours! Breaking your fast with a high-protein lunch will assist you in achieving your weight-loss objectives.

Steamed or grilled veggies can be combined with a range of proteins, including grilled beef, fish, pork, tofu, grains, eggs, nuts, legumes, and seeds, to name a few.

DAY 5

Task: 8h Eat | 16h Fast

Mission: Feeling hungry? Take coffee!

You'll eventually hit the ultimate 16/8 Intermittent Fasting regimen of fasting for 16 hours then feeding during an 8-hour timeframe on Day 5 of the Intermittent Fasting Plan. And it'll be relatively straightforward to do, as it is done by hundreds of individuals who have already achieved the 21-Day Intermittent Fasting Task.

It is suggested to drink black coffee to help you get through the 16-hour fast and curb your thirst. It's high in antioxidants and also works as an appetite suppressant. Keep in mind the coffee for Intermittent Fasting is dark. That is, no creamers, sugar, or milk— no latte, flat white, or cappuccino, just black coffee.

Are you a non-coffee drinker? Choose a bottle of water or a cup of black or green tea.

DAY 6

Task: 8h Eat | 16h Fast

Mission: Start walking

Are you planning to lose weight through these 21 days of fasting? Maintaining a balanced diet is important, and we also suggest adding exercise to your everyday routine.

Just before you leave your fast, go for a stroll. Even a short 20-minute stroll will suffice. Walking is an excellent way to boost your health, improve the attitude, and get some fresh air. Most notably, going on a stroll will distract you from your appetite and make the last few hours of fasting fly by faster.

DAY 7

Task: 8h Eat | 16h Fast

Mission: Keep walking

Maintain your current 16/8 Intermittent Fasting Schedule today and focus on your success from the previous week. Taking a full-body picture, tracking your weight, and comparing them to your initial weight and picture are all vital aspects of growth. Your body and physical features can start to change within a few weeks.

Chapter 2
Pro s and Cons of
Intermittent Fasting

Weight loss is possible with low-carb, high-fat (LCHF) diets, but we may be able to do even better with intermittent fasting, which has several advantages not available with traditional dieting. Both diets' goals are to enhance metabolic health, reduced insulin effect, and increase fat loss. Many people believe that eating too many calories causes weight gain, but this is only partly correct. Calories and insulin are most likely to blame for weight gain. LCHF diets not only lower insulin irrespective of calorie intake, but they also help you lose weight without even trying. As a result, LCHF is extremely effective for weight loss. Integrating fasting and LCHF, on the other hand, may provide a complimentary benefit for added benefit.

Weight reduction is achievable with LCHF diets, but we might be able to perform much more with intermittent fasting, which has a range of benefits not available through regular dieting. The aims of both diets are the same: to boost metabolic fitness, lower insulin effect, and increase fat loss. Most people assume that eating too many calories causes weight gain, although this is only partly true. Calories and insulin are most likely to blame for weight gain. LCHF diets not only reduce insulin levels independent of calorie intake, but they also help people lose weight without even trying. As a result, LCHF is highly beneficial for weight loss. Combining fasting and LCHF, on the other hand, could have a synergistic advantage for maximal impact.

Here are some advantages of fasting.

Simplicity

Although doctors may recommend that patients consume organic, locally raised grass-fed beef and skip white bread and packaged foods, the fact is that these food products are also ten times more costly. Simply put, some people cannot afford to eat properly. How come a pound of fresh cherries costs $6.99 and a whole loaf of bread costs $1.99? When you buy spaghetti and white bread, supporting a family on salary is a lot simpler. But that doesn't mean they have to live with type 2 diabetes and disease for the rest of their lives.

Fasting is a completely voluntary activity. It is not only free, but it also saves money since no food is needed. Except for saving money, nothing beats free. Who wouldn't want a few extra bucks in their wallet when losing weight and improving their health? It's as if you're being compensated for losing weight.

Convenience

It's nice to enjoy a home-cooked, made-from-scratch dinner, but many people don't have the time or ability to do so. Over the last two decades, the number of meals served outside of the household has grown. Despite the fact that many people want to help the "slow food revolution," it is clear that mainstream culture opposes the message. Cooking simply takes a long time. It's difficult to find time in jobs, blogging, and getting the kids to school and hockey. So, as honourable as it might be, telling people to dedicate themselves to home cooking is not a winning tactic for some.

On the other hand, fasting is the polar opposite. You save time when you are not ordering, buying, serving, or washing up food. It's a way to make your life easier.

Fasting simplifies your life where certain foods confuse it (eat this but not this, and just a little of the other). Why not save both time and money? It doesn't get any better than this.

Cheat days

Is it realistic to tell people that they can never, ever have ice cream again? For the rest of your life? Forever is a long time, and there will be celebrations. You can't consume dessert every day, but fasting encourages certain people to do so on occasion and while you feast, fasting tends to balance the scales. 'Cheat' days are valuable because they can help certain people develop enforcement for other days. While some people do well on an all-or-nothing strategy, fasting will help those who have been struggling with it for a long time balance their "cheat" days. The most critical part of fasting is integrating it into your everyday schedule.

Please note that we do not advocate "bingeing" and then "punishing" yourself. Instead, we believe that some people would do well with a little treat every now and then to balance out a fast easily.

Life has its ups and downs. There are ups and downs in everyone's life. There are days to look forward to and days to be feared. That's how it is. Some individuals, but not all, can benefit from an intermittent diet.

[Note: If you're hooked to sugar or other sweets, cheat days aren't a good idea. The all-or-nothing strategy fits well for certain people. Cheat days are not suggested for alcoholics, just as they are not advised for non-alcoholics.

It's tough to lose weight. All are aware of this. The most critical thing to pose for any nutritional adjustment is if it would succeed. The calorie-reduction diet of eating less and moving more seems like it should succeed, but does it? The majority of people will say no. Those diets perform wonders for some people while failing miserably for others. Diets will operate for a brief amount of time before stalling.

It also has virtually infinite capacity. What exactly does this imply? There is only one 'strength mode' on certain diets. What happens if you adopt the Mediterranean diet but don't lose weight? What steps would you take to become more 'Mediterranean'? There is just one power mode, and it is either on or off.

Since fasting is the easiest and most reliable way to lower insulin, it is almost universally successful. It is a different story. You can fast for ten hours or ten days (though we don't usually advocate long fasts, and if you do, make sure you're doing so under medical supervision).

You must, in the end, ask yourself this question. Do you think you'll lose weight if you don't eat anything for a week? Even an infant knows the importance of weight loss. It's almost certain to happen.

Which Is More Effective: Fasting or Low Carb?

There are only two more questions to be answered. First and foremost, is it harmful? In the opposite, there are major health advantages that may be recognized. Two, are you up to the challenge? Ok, you'll never know until you do it.

Flexibility

Fasting is possible at any place and at any time. You literally quit if you are not feeling good for some reason. It's fully reversible in a matter of minutes. Take into account bariatric surgery (stomach stapling).

These procedures are conducted so that people can fast for long periods of time. And, at least in the short term, they appear to work. However, these procedures have a high risk of complications, nearly all of these are permanent. There is no time limit.

You have the option of fasting for sixteen hours or sixteen days. There isn't a fixed timeline. You will fast heavily this week and not at all the next week.

It is subject to adjustment depending on the personal circumstances. Fasting can be done for any reason or for no reason at all. Why will we presume that someone who has never tried fasting for a week or a month cannot do so?

Add to any diet

What is the most important gain of all? Any diet can come in fasting. That's because fasting is what you don't do more than something you do. It's a subtraction problem, not an inclusion problem.

If you have any or more of the following conditions, you can still fast.

* You don't like meat, do you?

* You're not a wheat eater?

* Are you allergic to nuts?

* You don't have time to do it?

* You don't have any funds?

* Are you always on the move?

* You don't know how to cook?

* Are you above the age of 80?

* Do you have difficulty swallowing or chewing food?

It's that simple. It makes you save money. It helps you save time. Adaptable. Effortless. Available at any time and from any place. What might be more appealing than that?

Cells are repaired.

Since the body is not focused on food digestion, the repair mechanism is in full swing. It is able to focus entirely on cell repair. Autophagy is the term for this method.

Fasting thus assists in the regeneration or, in this case, the restoration of the body and its proper working.

Makes you see more clearly.

Another significant advantage of intermittent fasting is that you can concentrate better on assignments and complete a significant portion of your workload while fasting.

Helps to prevent insulin resistance.

Insulin tolerance develops as blood sugar levels are consistently elevated. It causes the body to be unable to respond to and break down the sugar content in your blood.

Intermittent fasting assists you with maintaining a healthy blood sugar intake. Elevated blood pressure, inactivity, biology, poor diet, obesity, or excess body weight may all contribute to this disorder.

Weight Loss

Intermittent fasting is often marketed as a weight-loss strategy that helps you to lose more weight while eating. Is that true, though? Intermittent fasting has been shown in studies to be an efficient way to reduce weight in both obese and non-obese people. Intermittent fasting, according to at least one study, can avoid metabolic down-regulation associated with weight loss by alternating periods of intense energy deficiency with periods of energy balance. As a result, it's likely that intermittent fasting, when opposed to other weight management strategies, would result in more consistent fat loss and better weight maintenance.

Other reports, however, have cast some doubt on this assumption, with one showing that alternate day fasting and steady caloric restriction achieved comparable weight loss outcomes. However, the alternate day fasting party in this sample had low enforcement, increasing the risk that the problem is more with adherence than with the biological mechanisms of fasting. Intermittent fasting has also been shown to increase diabetes markers and insulin sensitivity in other trials. Notably, the benefits were not solely due to weight loss; fasting seemed to improve cardiovascular fitness through specific fasting processes as well.

Fasting, in the end, is likely to cause weight loss solely or mostly by causing people to consume less. It's impossible not to lose weight if you reduce your daily meals from three to two.

It's difficult to know how much fasting lowers energy consumption because experiments almost all depend on participants self-reporting their food intake. However, weight loss is largely accomplished by eating less calories than you burn, according to research that have specifically tracked caloric consumption and expenditure.

Although it is commonly accepted that fasting extends one's life, this is impossible to establish in humans. The empirical evidence for fasting's longevity benefits is either direct, extrapolating from other health benefits of fasting, or it is indirect, based on animal studies (mostly mice and rats). To begin with, since fasting will help weight loss and avoid regaining weight, it would automatically prolong the lifetime of someone who is overweight. That aspect doesn't need much clarification. Fasting also encourages autophagy, a process that has been shown to lower cancer risk, prolong longevity, and increase general health in humans and several animals.

Fasting increases the lifetime of rodents, fruit flies, rats, primates, and other small animals, according to studies; however, since this question cannot be explicitly tested in humans, the question of whether fasting per se has longevity effects for humans remains unanswered.

Intermittent fasting tends to enhance digestive quality in different animal species, both by effects on the gut and effects on the gut microbiota, according to a growing body of proof. However, the effect isn't uniform for all primates, and further research into how fasting impacts human gut health is needed.

Intermittent fasting tends to prolong human lifespan via a combination of weight loss and decreased risk of cancer and neurodegenerative disease through autophagy, although other pathways, such as gut wellbeing, remain unclear and need to be investigated in humans.

2.2 Drawbacks of Intermittent Fasting

Here are a few issues that might come up in the first few months of intermittent fasting.

No weight loss

You could be maintaining water weight even if you've never lost the weight in a few days. That can't go on indefinitely. You can either wait it out or enable rapid water weight loss by reducing carbohydrates & sodium intake.

If you haven't lost some weight in two weeks or more, you're simply eating too much. Reduce your fat and carb intake, increase your lean protein & vegetable intake, and drink plenty of water.

If you're losing weight too fast

It's the opposite of the previous object, with the exception that it's much more probable to be water weight. You'll lose the weight quickly if you limit your salt consumption, sugars, and food in general. Most of it would be water weight and the components of your stomach; no one loses multiple pounds of fat in a single day.

Take stock of your fitness and energy level if you ever feel like you're losing the weight "too quickly." You're likely not dropping weight too quickly if you're feeling healthy. Obese people can lose weight much quicker and comfortably with a high enough calorie deficit, even though two pounds per week is frequently touted as a guideline.

If you want to reduce speed your weight loss, increase your daily calorie intake by two to three hundred calories, preferably from high-protein foods like beans, eggs, beef, or tofu.

Afternoon energy crashes

Some people have recurring energy slumps at certain times of the day, typically in the afternoon. This can be caused by several factors.

To begin with, you might not be eating a proper breakfast. Make it a little bit bigger.

Second, if you don't eat carbs for breakfast, you could go into ketosis and get the keto flu. Although you don't want to start your day with a high-carb meal, it's always a good idea to eat at least 10 to 20 grams of carbohydrates to prevent draining your glycogen stores and experiencing ketosis.

Finally, caffeine could be causing you to crash. To make missing breakfast easier, many people increase their caffeine intake in the morning. When you're a caffeine addict, consider halving your daily dose.

Low blood sugar

If you're experiencing constant nausea, headaches, or dizziness while on the IF diet, it's a red flag that your blood sugar is out of whack. People with diabetes can stop fasting diets for the following reasons, as previously stated by WH: Hypoglycaemia, a serious incident for those with thyroid or insulin disorders, may be caused by IF.

Insomnia

Hunger, a shortage of carbohydrates, or caffeine are the most common causes of insomnia on an IF diet.

If you're a caffeine consumer, consider cutting your caffeine consumption in half, as previously mentioned. When it comes to the first two, you might consider switching your eating window back an hour and adding 30 extra grams of carbs to your final meal of the day. Almost always, either or both would suffice.

Food cravings

Intermittent fasting does not cause you to adjust what you feed, only when you eat it. Cravings for food can occur because you're starving, but they're generally psychological in nature.

Food cravings will be satisfied for a short time, but they will become greater in the long run if they are fed. The easiest way to deal with food cravings is to ignore them and stick to your diet plan. The better it gets when your food cravings disappear, the more you stick to your diet.

That said, you probably would not like to give up your favourite foods - that's great - but you do need to set limits on when you can eat them, so it doesn't become "whenever you feel like it." Allowing yourself to eat "junk" foods during your post-workout meal is the perfect time to do so. It works on a physical level by providing calories to your muscles, and it also works on a psychological level by inspiring you to exercise.

According to Koens, being on a restricted diet may influence your relationship with food. While some people love the strictness of IF, others can find themselves obsessing about when they should eat and how much calories they're eating.

Spending too much time every day worrying about the quantity or quality of your food can lead to orthorexia, a form of eating disorder. Orthorexia is a condition in which you place such a high value on "right" or "healthy" eating that it has a negative impact on your overall health.

According to Koens, the aim of any diet should be to form a safe, meaningful relationship with food, not to lose weight.

Hair Loss

Is this for real? Yes. Hair loss can be caused by sudden losing weight or a lack of adequate nutrients, particularly protein and B vitamins, according to Koens.

Although intermittent fasting (IF) does not always result in nutritional loss, it is more difficult to eat a well-balanced diet when you're cramming a full day's worth of eating into a few hours. If you notice more hair falling out in the shower than normal, re-evaluate the nutritional quality of your regular meals and consult with your doctor about whether IF is a good fit for you.

Irritable bowel syndrome

Is all backed up? It's possible that IF is to blame. "If you don't get enough fluid, vitamins, protein, or fibre, any diet can cause an upset stomach," says Koens, who stresses the importance of keeping hydrated during the day.

People sometimes forget to drink water during fasting hours, she says, but going 16 hours with little fluid is a recipe for tragedy (gastrointestinal). So, if you've started an IF diet and aren't having normal bowel movements, it's time to put your plan on hold and talk to a nutritionist or doctor about what's going on.

Sleep disturbances

Many people report better sleep patterns when doing IF, according to Koens, probably because IF helps curb late-night snacking behaviours, which can lead to an unwillingness to fall asleep while your stomach is still digesting the 10 p.m. snack.

However, some evidence indicates that the opposite is true. Evidence suggests that intermittent diurnal fasting (daytime fasting) reduces rapid-eye-movement (REM) sleep, according to a study published in the journal Nature and Science of Sleep in 2018. According to the Harvard Business Review, getting enough REM sleep has been related to a variety of health benefits, including improved memory, cognitive processing, and attention. It's unclear why this is the case.

If you're having trouble falling or staying asleep after beginning an IF eating plan, pause and consult a specialist to ensure you're not damaging your health.

Traveling

When you're on the road, you'll have to be a bit more flexible with your schedule. Enable for a four- to nine-hour eating window and a 14- to 24-hour fasting window on days when you travel through time zones.

You can need to be more versatile in terms of what you eat as well. Nut bags are typically used in airports and are a nice choice. In the end, breaking the rules a little for a day is perfect. If you don't eat out or eat fast food. It's good to eat a sandwich on a low-carb diet, for example.

Frequent flyers, on the other hand, would need to be cautious about this because they fly often enough to make it a concern. However, most people would be happy with a day of violating the rules here now and there if the circumstances really warrant it.

Chapter 3
Types of
Intermittent Fasting

Intermittent fasting can be achieved in a variety of ways. The choice of fasting styles is primarily based on personal preference and the ease with which you can stick to a given fasting schedule, as studies have not specifically tested the beneficial effects of one over the other.

3.1 16/8 Fasting

THE 16/8 METHOD							
	DAY 1	DAY 2	DAY 3	DAY 4	DAY 5	DAY 6	DAY 7
Midnight 4 AM 8 AM	FAST	FAST	FAST	FAST	FAST	FAST	FAST
12 PM	First meal	First meal	First meal	First meal	First meal	First meal	First meal
4 PM	Last meal by 8pm	Last meal by 8pm	Last meal by 8pm	Last meal by 8pm	Last meal by 8pm	Last meal by 8pm	Last meal by 8pm
8 PM Midnight	FAST	FAST	FAST	FAST	FAST	FAST	FAST

Martin Berkhan of Leangains made the 16/8 fasting method popular and it is still the most prevalent intermittent fasting plan. As the name implies, this method includes 16 hours of fasting daily with eight-hour window to eat.

This plan is successful because it is simple to follow on a daily basis and creates a perfect balance between dietary restriction, adherence ease, and consistency. Many people miss breakfast, and their eating window is between noon and 8 p.m., or even later. This is perhaps the most "lifestyle friendly" choice for many people because eating in the evening makes it much easier to sleep, and many people do find that fasting in the morning keeps them very focused throughout the workday.

Another benefit of this schedule is that it becomes routine; after a few days, you won't be hungry during the fasting time, especially when you are fasting in the morning.

The 16/8 fasting method is undoubtedly the simplest way to begin intermittent fasting, and it is frequently the very first intermittent fasting method that people have tried.

3.2 19/5 FASTING

19/5 fasting is similar to 16/8 fasting in concept, but it limits the feeding window to five hours. A 19/5 fasting method lets you take precisely two meals per day at the start and end of the feeding window, while 16/8 fasting allows for around two to three meals per day.

Although the 19/5 fasting schedule seems to be close to the 16/8 fasting schedule, it may be considerably more difficult for many people to adhere to. It's partially due to hunger, but it's more likely due to the fact that this schedule causes people to skip family dinners - unlike the 16/8 schedule, there's no way to eat lunch and dinner on this schedule.

On the plus side, by limiting yourself to two meals a day and leaving no time for snacking between those, you'll be able to lose weight much more quickly.

3.3 One meal a day

The one meal a day fasting method is perhaps the most intense daily fasting schedule. It is not really well known, and most people find it incredibly hard, but some people firmly express their confidence in it.

The benefits are equivalent to those of the 19/5 easy, but they are more obvious. On this plan, it's practically impossible to gain weight.

This routine, on the other hand, will make it tough to eat healthy food, in addition to having an effect on your lifestyle. And besides, during this plan several people should consume around 1500 to 3000 calories in a single meal. You may as well not try this program if you can't do it without eating fast food to gain calories.

3.4 Occasional 24–48-hour fasts

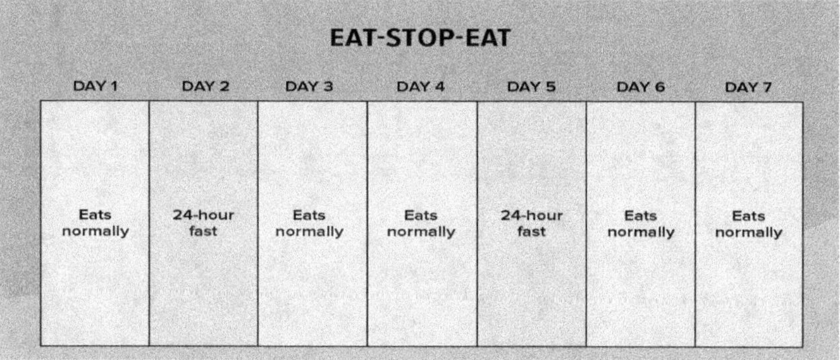

Many people fast for one to two days per week or month, shifting away from fasting every day. The key benefits of this fasting method are that it allows quick fat loss during the fasting time, and that even fasting for 24 hours per month is enough to avoid steady fat gain while also improving cardiovascular health.

There is also some research proof that increasing autophagy requires you to fast for 24-48 hours, indicating that this plan could be preferable to shortened daily fasts for longer lifespan.

Most people believe that this method is more helpful than fasting on a regular basis, but many do not. In this case, the real disadvantage is that, as with a regular daily fast, your appetite never truly adjusts; you might feel starved during your fasting period if you do this.

A 24-hour fast spans from previous night dinner to the dinner next day, the night of the fast. A 36-hour fast spans from the dinner of previous night, whole day fast and then before the breakfast of the next morning. A 48-hour fast spans from one dinner, fasting the two days till the dinner of second day.

Fasting for 24 hours takes some getting used to, but it is possible. Fasting for 36 hours is normally more difficult since it is difficult to sleep while fasted. Fasting for 48 hours is daunting for almost all and can be performed only about once a month at the most.

3.5 The 5:2 Method

THE 5:2 DIET

DAY 1	DAY 2	DAY 3	DAY 4	DAY 5	DAY 6	DAY 7
Eats normally	Women: *500 calories* Men: *600 calories*	Eats normally	Eats normally	Women: *500 calories* Men: *600 calories*	Eats normally	Eats normally

This fasting approach includes eating regularly every five days a week and limiting calorie consumption to 500-600 calories for the rest of two days (not consecutively). Women should consume approximately 500 calories on fasting days, and men must consume approximately 600 calories.

ALTERNATE-DAY FASTING

DAY 1	DAY 2	DAY 3	DAY 4	DAY 5	DAY 6	DAY 7
Eats normally	24-hour fast OR Eat only a few hundred calories	Eats normally	24-hour fast OR Eat only a few hundred calories	Eats normally	24-hour fast OR Eat only a few hundred calories	Eats normally

Alternate-day fasting is when people fast for 24 to 36 hours more than once every week. People fast every other day while on this plan. Then, on consuming days, they can eat whatever they want. On fasting days, the feeding window is usually 24 hours, which means people take a healthy dinner just before going to bed.

Because consuming double as much food on eating days is incredibly difficult, this plan inevitably leads to weight loss even while not on a diet. It also is easier to adapt to than you would expect - but by no means easy.

For weight loss and cardiovascular health, alternate day fasting (ADF) is at least as successful as daily food restriction. Despite the fact that the approach used in that research was faulty, another study found it to be more efficient - food was given to the ADF group but not to the daily food restriction group.

If ADF is easier, it's more probably due to the fact that it's more difficult to overeat and not know it on this diet, instead of any physical gain.

3.7 Longer-term fasts

Intermittent fasting is not defined as a period of fasting that lasts longer than 48 hours. Fasting has traditionally been performed for religious or protest reasons, but an increasing number of people have begun fasting for prolonged periods of time in order to improve their lives.

This is not supported by research. Apart from the basic issues of adherence, muscle atrophy, and metabolic downregulation, recent study showed that autophagy rises around 24 and 48 hours and then starts to decrease after that. There really is such a concern as too much autophagy; it is not really a matter of "the more, the better."

With this in sight, it is probably best to fast for 24-48 hours on a regular basis instead of just doing prolonged fasts on occasion.

3.8 Regular vs. ad hoc fasting

The majority of people fast on a routine basis, such as every day starting from 8 p.m. to noon or every Sunday till 9 p.m.

Some people, on the other hand, fast without keeping to a rigid schedule, preferring to fast anytime their schedule allows them - for instance, a 24-hour fast if they get a day free of social responsibilities, or 16-hour fasts a few times a week.

Either approach will suffice; there is no need to fast on a daily basis in order to take full advantage. Fasting on ad hoc basis, on the other hand, is not always convenient, despite the fact that it provides more freedom.

It is tough, if not impossible, to develop new habits when you do not adhere to a schedule. You will feel hungrier during your fasting times because your body does not really change its appetite to accommodate the fasting schedule.

As a result, it is recommended that you adhere to a fixed fasting routine for at least the first two months of the fasting to develop a fasting routine. Afterwards, if you want to, you should try out ad hoc fasting.

3.9 Spontaneous Meal Skipping

SPONTANEOUS MEAL SKIPPING

	DAY 1	DAY 2	DAY 3	DAY 4	DAY 5	DAY 6	DAY 7
	Breakfast	Skipped Meal	Breakfast	Breakfast	Breakfast	Breakfast	Breakfast
	Lunch	Lunch	Lunch	Lunch	Lunch	Lunch	Lunch
	Dinner	Dinner	Dinner	Dinner	Skipped Meal	Dinner	Dinner

If you are not really hungry, miss meals.

And if you do eat, adhere to your regular eating schedule.

This fasting diet takes an intelligent approach, making it suitable for those looking for ultimate convenience. In non-fasting hours, eat a diet containing minimum carbohydrates and high-quality fats, such as that of the keto diet, to maintain a healthy lifestyle, keep your blood sugar levels stable, and even prolong your fasting time.

Chapter 4
How to Start 16/8
Intermittent Fasting

It is simple to get going, but not as simple as getting started right now. It's best to schedule ahead of time, much like anything else in life. In five basic steps, and here is the how to get started.

4.1 Step one: Plan your eating window around your schedule

While most people eat between noon to 8:00 pm or similar to that, the feeding time can be any 8 hours that you're awake.

There are some things to think about while picking an eating window:

Sleep is helped by feeding in the evening, carbohydrates in particular. Aside from the apparent fact that it's difficult to sleep while you're starving, carbohydrates are often used by your brain to manufacture serotonin, which is a key to melatonin. Check out my full guide to insomnia for more details on sleep.

It's easier to keep a healthy social life if you have both lunch as well as dinner in your dining window. If you must choose between two, dinner usually takes priority.

You'll actually be more emotionally aware during your fasting time after a few days of acclimating to fasting. It has the ability to improve productivity.

You can eat before and after your workout - see the next section for more details.

Consider what you eat in relation to your daily routine - for most people that work 9-5, this means breakfast at 8:00 a.m., lunch at 12:00 p.m., and dinner at 6:00 p.m. You may include whether breakfast or dinner in that case, but not both.

Although I've mentioned this as the first move, you may want to start with the next thing - choosing when you'll workout - and then settle on a diet plan. It all relies as to which of the 2 you have much more control over. If you just have a certain amount of time to exercise, you can schedule your workout first and then your eating window.

After examining the list of factors above, it's easy to see why the hours between noon and 8 p.m. are so common for dining. It crosses all the boxes, meaning you can exercise in that time period and more assuming you have a fairly normal schedule, running anywhere between 9 and 5.

You have some leeway in terms of what you eat. You can change it up to 2 hours in any direction on any specific day as a general rule, but you shouldn't do it more than two times a week. It's also fine to break it down a little - render eight hours the limit and five hours the minimum.

4.2 STEP TWO: DETERMINE WHEN YOU'LL EXERCISE

It's better not to work out on an empty stomach because your workout requires calories as well as protein to be successful. While you're doing resistance training (lifting weights, you'll would like to eat either one or two meals afterward to help your muscles develop.

With this in mind, you can exercise near the start of your diet plan, right after you've broken your fast. If that isn't practical, try to train during your eating window's middle hours.

If you have to exercise at the end of your eating window, receive a decent post-workout meal or snack - even if it's just a protein bar or shake - to help with recovery and muscle work out growth.

Although you likely won't work out each day, it's still better to stick to the same meal plan every day instead of attempting to differentiate between exercise and rest days for habit-building purposes.

You can schedule your mealtimes within your diet plan and related to your exercise time when you have a diet and an exercise time.

4.3 STEP THREE: DETERMINE MEALTIMES

You'll need to find out particular mealtimes once you've developed an overall eating window as well as an exercise period. If you have an eight-hour window, you'll consume 2 meals, 3 meals, or 2 meals and 1 snack.

Here's an illustration of a typical scenario: someone prefers the approximately noon to eight windows however pushes it back a little to suit their timetable.

* Working hours: 8:00 a.m. to 5:00 p.m.

* Time of eating: 1-9 p.m.

* 1-2 p.m. for the first meal

* 5-5:30 p.m.: Snack or secondary meal

* Workout time is 5:30 p.m.

* Dinner is served from 7:30-8:30 p.m.

As you can see, having a late lunch allows this person to go to the gym after work, eat before as well as after their exercise, and has enough time among meals and workouts to not feel hurried.

4.4 STEP FOUR: DETERMINE MEAL COMPOSITION

Intermittent fasting does not necessitate a strict diet besides the fasting itself. Regardless, you should have an idea of what you'll eat and when you'll eat it.

Based on your dieting style, it might mean that you have large calorie expectations to every meal or just a basic understanding of what types of foods you'll eat. Here are some pointers to think about:

Daily protein consumption of 6 grams per pound of body weight. Make it if you're overweight. Instead, eight grams per pound of lean mass.

Protein should be distributed uniformly during the day, with the first meal being marginally higher in protein.

Every meal should involve at least Five grams of fat; otherwise, fat timing is unimportant.

Carbohydrates should be consumed later in the day, in the meal immediately after a workout.

At minimum 1 serving of fruits and vegetables should be included with every meal, and you should aim for 5 servings of vegetables and 3 servings of fruit per day.

Since higher-calorie meals can cause you to become exhausted, meals should be larger in the evening.

If you consume the same few items for most meals, especially the earlier ones, it's very easier to develop stable habits. For the most part, giving yourself further variety in the last meal is the best choice.

Here's how the individual in the preceding example will likely schedule their meals based on those guidelines:

* Service hours are from 8 a.m. to 5 p.m.

* Time to eat: 1-9 p.m.

* 1-2 p.m.: First meal. A small, high-protein, low-carb meal. On weekdays, a burrito dish or chicken salad is usually consumed near the workplace; on weekends, bacon, eggs, fruits, and vegetables are consumed at home.

* 5-5:30 p.m.: Snack or second meal-either a protein bar or even a small sandwich.

* 5:30 p.m.: Workout

* Dinner will be served between 7:30 and 8:30 p.m.

A big high-carb dinner, like pasta or pie, on gym days. A lighter, relatively high-carb breakfast, including a stir fry with potatoes, on most days.

4.5 Step five: Start fasting, and track your meals

It's time to begin now that you've sorted out everything. For a minimum of the first 2 months, use a diet tracker like MyFitnessPal to keep track of your meals, even mealtimes.

If you're serious about it and get started right away, you'll find yourself in a comfortable rhythm within the first week. You'll feel hungry just before your regular meal hours, and you'll feel less hungry after your fasting period.

4.6 Tips to Make Intermittent Fasting Easier

1. Drink Plenty of Water

To further eliminate any cravings, squeeze a little either lemon or lime juice into your water. You should also consume calorie-free drinks like coffee or tea. Within a couple weeks, you'll notice that intermittent fasting completely eliminates your sugar cravings.

2. Take in Caffeine in the Morning and Early Afternoon

Caffeine in coffee as well as tea will help you lose weight by curbing your appetite, making intermittent fasting a bit easier. Take note not to overindulge, because this could make you feel a little jittery. These organic energy-boosting tips are also advised to keep you working during the day.

3. Avoid Artificially Flavoured Drinks

Diet sodas and other drinks containing artificial sweeteners such as Splenda and Sweet & Low should be avoided as calorie-free beverages. According to studies, they will increase your appetite in the same way as a sugary soda can, causing you to overeat.

4. Don't Gorge at Your First Meal

After your fast, your first meal ought to be the amount of food you usually consume. Binging might only make you feel worse and negate the advantages of your fast.

Create menu schedules, at minimum for the first few weeks, to prevent this. It will assist you in developing a regimen of regularly portioned meals throughout your eating window.

5. Minimize Processed Carbohydrates and Sugars

Although intermittent fasting allows you to consume just that little looser than usual, you can also consume as little rice, pasta, bread, and other carbohydrates as possible.

Instead, eat protein-rich foods like meat, chicken, and pork, as well as carbs like vegetables, berries, and sweet potatoes, and healthier fats like fish, avocados, almonds, and olive oil.

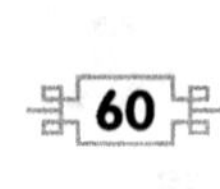

Chapter 5
When to Avoid
Intermittent Fasting
(as a Woman Over 50)

The intermittent fasting is not recommended in certain cases, according to health experts. In this chapter, we have looked at a few examples of this. If any of the following situations applies to you, you should refrain from fasting intermittently unless otherwise advised.

5.1 Sleep Problems

Sleep is important for recovering and healing muscles after exercise, promoting brain activity, and even preserving emotional well-being. Heading to sleep hungry will make it difficult for your body to get relaxed and fall asleep because it triggers your brain to become alert, causing your body to become restless. Sass adds her two cents: "If the end of their IF eating window is far too early in the day, I've had clients struggle to fall asleep or stay asleep. Sleep deprivation poses a range of health hazards, since it is during this period that your body heals and repairs itself."

Moreover, if you do not eat for several hours, the sugar levels of your blood may eventually drop, causing you to wake up feeling nervous from your deep sleep. Disturbance in sleep can be dangerous to the health, particularly if they happen during the most important stage of sleep — the rapid eye movement (REM) sleep cycle.

This stage is critical for remembering and storing knowledge learned throughout the day, and it occurs many times in your sleep. Of course, not getting enough sleep will lead to other issues, such as being unable to remember things.

"Insufficient sleep will affect weight control and pose a safety risk with regard to cognitive functioning and driving," Sass says. IF is not really helping you shed pounds in this situation, but it is one of the reasons that make you gain weight.

5.2 Eating Disorders

"Disordered eating is used to characterize a variety of abnormal eating habits which might or might not require a diagnosis of a particular eating disorder," as per the Academy of Nutrition and Dietetics. Rather than being a diagnosis, disordered eating is defined as a descriptive term. If abnormal eating patterns and behaviours are not treated, an eating disorder including anorexia nervosa, bulimia nervosa, or emotional eating may develop. Intermittent fasting, according to Sass, may not be the right solution for someone who has suffered with eating disorders or unhealthy eating habits.

"In people with this background, any approach that promotes restraint can lead to a disordered pattern. It's vital for everyone, but especially for anyone with this past, to listen to their bodies and be aware of what makes them feel good emotionally and physically. If restricting your calorie intake doesn't help you do this, you're on the wrong track" she declares.

5.3 INTENSE EXERCISE

Trying to do intermittent fasting when participating in an intensive training period is not an appropriate or healthy combination, as one might expect.

If you have been practicing to participate in a marathon or do Strength training on a daily basis, you might want to think twice about doing IF. To assist you get through your training, you would have to eat a little before you begin. Moreover, it is indeed important to consume enough food once you have completed your workout. "You may damage your muscle tissues and drain your glycogen reserves during a hard workout," informs Kacie Vavrek, RD, a sports medicine practicing dietitian at The Ohio State University Wexner Medical Centre. "A replenishing meal after one or two hours, followed by daily meals around 3-4 hours, would aid in restocking glycogen reserves and repairing and rebuilding muscle during the day," says the author. According to Vavrek, missing this meal after a workout will slow your healing and even prevent important muscle growth and recovery.

And likewise, if we assume that you are attempting to increase your muscle mass, as well in this case, Sass recommends that you should eat protein at various times during the day instead of attempting to fit everything into a single eating window. According to many studies, the body cannot effectively digest more than 1-1.2 in of protein in a single meal. As a result, all extra protein eaten throughout the day that is not used during exercising and weightlifting is stored as fat rather than muscle.

"Dividing protein intake during the day and having a protein-rich snack around an hour before sleeping" are two research-backed methods to help you grow muscle mass. "This strategy is countered by limiting the eating window to only eight hours," Sass continues.

"Nutritional scheduling is necessary for athletic success and will be difficult to achieve on an IF diet," confirms Allison Knott, MS, RDN, CSSD, a nutrition expert in New York City.

"Due to the extra calories consumed, endurance sports involve higher calorie requirements. To regenerate muscle, replenish glycogen reserves, and preserve electrolyte balance, endurance exercise generally requires regular calorie intake and sufficient macronutrient intake prior, during, then after an exercise or lengthy training."

Intermittent fasting does not provide you with the consistent supply of nutrients and energy that you need to practice, exercise, and heal. If you're planning on participating in an endurance event, you should stop intermittent fasting.

5.4 Digestive problems

If stomach problems were not bad enough, throwing a messed-up eating routine further into equation would just make it worse. "If you have history of digestive issues (such as IBS), intermittent fasting can intensify your problems," Calder advises.

Given the long fasting periods, IF can indeed trigger gastrointestinal issues. "Fasting periods may interrupt the digestive system's normal functions, resulting in constipation, acid reflux, and indigestion."

Huge meals, which are often needed for IF that entails a long fast, can also cause digestive distress, according to Bannan. "This would be especially troubling for individuals with IBS, who have a sensitive gut already," she says.

5.5 Focused/Hard Job

Food offers nourishment and stamina, as well as the ability to concentrate. If you're very hungry, the most you can think of is food, which takes your focus away from the job at hand. Certainly, everybody reacts to IF in a different manner - it varies person to person - but when you are not used to enduring extended periods without food, it can impair your ability to focus initially.

"While some people have experienced increased energy levels as a result of intermittent fasting, someone else can encounter weakness, decreased focus, and loss of energy,"

Calder states. "It will have an effect on your everyday productivity. If you work in a job or do things that take a great deal of energy and focus, intermittent fasting might not be the best choice for you."

5.6 Diabetes

"If you are already diabetic and therefore are taking diabetes medications, particularly insulin, you should not be doing intermittent fasting before consulting a physician and being carefully monitored," recommends Calder. "When intermittent fasting is paired with diabetes medicines, blood sugar levels can drop critically low."

Calder goes so far as to suggest that someone with low blood sugar problems must skip IF since they need to eat regularly to keep their blood sugar levels steady.

"Intermittent fasting is a form of fasting that alternates between fasting periods and unrestricted eating periods. This may be extremely hazardous for diabetes patients who use anti-diabetic drugs, particularly insulin "Endocrinologist and creator of New York Endocrinology, Dr. Rocio Salas-Whalen, confirms.

"On fasting days, anti-diabetic prescriptions, especially insulin, can continue to affect blood sugar levels. It has the potential to cause dangerously low blood sugar levels."

To stay healthy, people with diabetes must keep their blood sugar levels stable (with both exercise and diet). With intermittent fasting, it becomes almost unlikely.

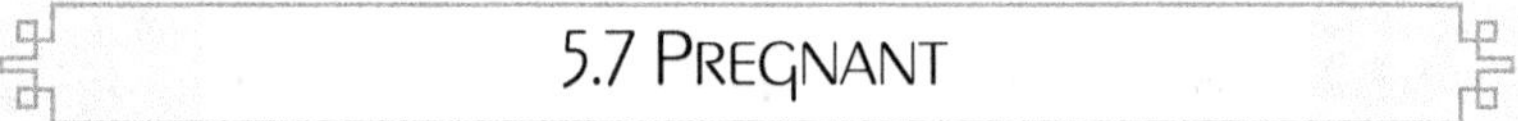

5.7 PREGNANT

IF may be harmful to a child's growth if done while pregnant or breastfeeding. According to Calder, "Pregnancy and breastfeeding necessarily involve a sufficient calorie intake in order for the baby to grow effectively and for milk production to occur. Intermittent fasting can clash with your daily calories, so it is not recommended for pregnant or breastfeeding women."

While you are trying to have a baby, IF might not be the best option for you. According to Bannan, IF has been related to fertility problems, as well as changes in menstruation, metabolism, and even cause early menopause in females.

To ensure the health of your baby and yourself, during pregnancy, you will need to eat a maternity diet rich in nutrients and calories. You will not have it with intermittent fasting, unfortunately.

"Intermittent fasting is not recommended for chronically ill people such as diabetics or cancer patients because it can result in low blood sugar, insufficient calorie intake, and inability to meet nutritional needs. This is also applicable to pregnant and lactating women, who have higher calorie and nutrient requirements" Knott confirms.

When you are pregnant, you will have to eat frequently and in adequate amounts to maintain your and your child's safety. That is not possible given the arrangement of intermittent fasting.

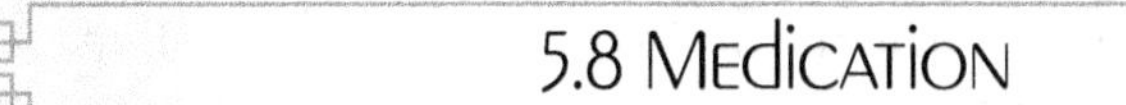

5.8 Medication

Some drugs must be consumed with food as, among other things, they may leave you feeling dizzy and nauseous if you take them on an empty stomach. People who have to take a number of supplements or vitamins per day can be affected by IF fasting cycles.

Anyone with anaemia or an iron deficiency in their blood, for instance, can need to take one or several iron pills every day to maintain the normal iron levels. Iron supplements are known to cause nausea and having them with meals will help to alleviate this experience. Although taking an iron supplement at any time of day is possible, but when you're on a medicine which can only be taken at a particular time and also with food? This is when things start to really get complicated, and it's certainly not a good idea to start this diet when it doesn't fit with your medicine.

5.9 Weak Immune System

Many who have previously undergone or are currently experiencing a terminal disease should not indulge in IF before even consulting their doctor. Because: "Sufficient caloric intake is required in several cases to retain lean muscle mass and a strong immune system, that is important for people with cancer or compromised immune systems," advises Calder. "Before initiating intermittent fasting, such patients should consult with a doctor." To boost your immune system response, avoid IF and add healthier habits to your routine.

5.10 Tough Schedule

Your daily work routine may have a significant role to play in order participate in IF regime effectively. What are you doing, for instance, if you work overnight and must sleep throughout the day, however one of your feeding intervals occurs during the day? Worse than that, what about when the most of your fast take place during work? What about if you practice different shifts every day and do not have a regular schedule? Fasting periods, according to Bannan, will leave you feeling cold, cause headaches, and cause mood swings. Having to put up with all these other possible side effects could cause you to lose concentration and productivity at work.

Chapter 6
Intermittent Fasting Recipes for Women Over 50

6.1 Ginger Chili Beef with Tender stem

Preparation time 45 minutes | Servings 2 persons | Nutritional facts 240 calories

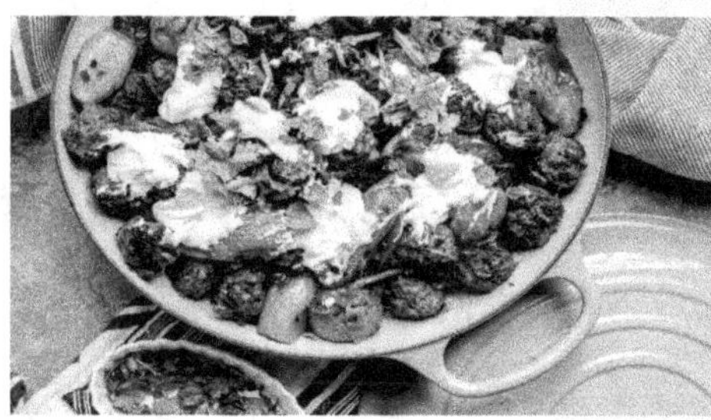

Ingredients

*   ½ finely sliced red pepper

*   1 red chili, de-seeded

*   1 sirloin steak piece of about 10,5 oz

*   1 sliced thickly bunch of spring onions

*   1 tbsp fresh coriander, chopped

* 1 tbsp of soy sauce

* 3,5 oz baby corn, lengthways halved

* 0,8 in peeled root ginger piece

* 2 handfuls beansprouts

* 2 peeled garlic cloves

* 2 strips of cooked rice noodles

* 2 tbsp dry sherry or rice wine

* 2 tbsp of runny honey

* 2 tbsp wok/stir-fry oil

* 7 oz tender stem, halved

* 2,6 oz bamboo shoots

INSTRUCTIONS

The specific rules for preparing this delicious meal for women over 50 can be found below. These instructions must be followed in the order specified.

* Put the beef steak in a tray and trim away any excess fat before cutting it into wafer-thin strips.

* Using your hands or a handheld food processor, finely cut the garlic, chilli, and ginger. Stir into the beef strips and leave to marinate for thirty minutes at room temperature.

* In a broad wok, heat one tablespoon of oil. When the pan is nearly smoking, add the beef and marinade and stir-fry for a few minutes, or until the meat is cooked and golden. Remove the pan from the heat and place it somewhere warm to keep it warm.

* Return the wok to the heat with the remaining one tablespoon of oil. Place the tender stem, baby corn, and red pepper in the pan until it is almost smoking. Stir-fry for a few minutes, or until the vegetables soften. Before adding the beef and noodles, stir in the bean sprouts, bamboo shoots, and string onions for about a minute. Cook the noodles in a pan until they are completely cooked.

* In a mixing bowl, combine the honey, sherry, and soy sauce. Cook for one minute in the pan, flipping it around to cover it in sauce, and then serve. Serve with a coriander garnish.

6.2 CANTONESE GARLIC KING PRAWN

Preparation time 12-15 minutes | Servings 2 persons | Nutritional facts 240 calories

INGREDIENTS

* 1 green pepper, finely diced

* 1 medium white onion, finely diced

* 1/2 tsp salt

* 1/4 tsp white pepper

* 16 large raw king prawns

* 1 tsp sugar

* 2 tbsp vegetable oil

* 4 tbsp salted butter

* 5 garlic cloves, finely grated and chopped

The step-by-step instructions for preparing this nutritious meal for women over 50 can be found below. These instructions must be followed in the order specified.

* Cut a slit down to the back of every prawn to eliminate the digestion. After washing under cool water and draining, set aside.

* Heat the wok to medium-high. When the pan is hot, Put the oil & swirl it around to steam it up before adding the diced onion and cooking for thirty seconds.

* Fry for another 20 seconds after adding the garlic. Insert the green pepper and the entire drained king prawns after 30 seconds.

* Stir-fry for an additional two minutes, or until the prawns are pink.

* Generously season the fat with the salt, pepper, and sugar.

* Cook for 2-3 minutes longer, or when the prawns are fully cooked. Serve with a smile on your face.

6.3 PAYSAN BRETON SALMON & HORSERADISH TARTS

Preparation time 30 minutes | Servings 4 persons | Nutritional facts 240 calories

INGREDIENTS

* 1 tub Paysan Breton French Garlic & Herb cream cheese (5,3 oz)

* 3,5 oz smoked salmon, roughly chopped

* 2 tsp horseradish

* 7 oz spinach

* 13,2 oz pack ready-rolled puff pastry

* Freshly ground black pepper

* Zest of half a lemon

INSTRUCTIONS

The detailed instructions for making this wonderful meal for women over 50 can be found below. These directives must be followed in the order specified.

* Preheat the oven to 350 degrees Fahrenheit.

* Unroll the puff pastry, use a fifteen-centimetre circular cutter to cut out four triangles, and place on a parchment-lined baking sheet.

* Poke the pastry all over with a fork, then bake for 5-6 minutes, or until puffed and golden.

* Blanch the spinach for 1-2 minutes in salted water, or until wilted. Drain and set the water aside to cool. Once it has cooled, squeeze out any residual moisture.

* In a large mixing cup, add the cream cheese, horseradish, smoked salmon, spinach, and lemon zest.

* Season to perfection with freshly ground black pepper.

* Spread half of the cream cheese mixture into each pastry shell, leaving a border around the edges.

* Bake for an additional 5-6 minutes, just until the topping is golden brown and piping hot.

* Eat instantly and enjoy.

6.4 Peanut butter cookies

Preparation time 17 minutes | Servings 18 cookies |
Nutritional facts 240 calories

Ingredients

* 1 cup peanut butter

* 1 cup sugar

* 1 egg

Instructions

The specific rules for making this wonderful meal for women over 50 can be found below. These directives must be followed in the order specified.

* Preheat oven to 350 degrees Fahrenheit.

* In a large mixing cup, add all of the ingredients and stir until smooth. Scoop onto a parchment-lined baking sheet. (If you don't have a spoon, use your hands to roll the dough into one-inch balls.) Push down with the back of the fork to create the criss-cross shape on top. Then click in the same direction once more.

* There will be no spreading of these cookies. You can bake the whole recipe on a single baking tray if you want. Bake for 12 minutes, then cool on the tray for 1-2 minutes before switching to a wire rack to cool entirely. They should be kept in an airtight jar.

* Three ingredients are what you need to make buttery shortbread cookies.

6.5 Delicious Homemade cookies

Preparation time 45 minutes | Servings 3 dozen | Nutritional facts 128 calories

Ingredients

* 1 cup packed light brown sugar

* 2 cups salted butter, cold and cut into pieces

* 4 1/2 cups all-purpose flour, divided

Optional: Your favourite sprinkles

Instructions

The specific rules for making this wonderful meal for women over 50 can be found below. These directives must be followed in the order specified.

* Preheat the oven to 325 degrees Fahrenheit and place the rack in the lower-middle spot.

* The first move is to line baking sheets with parchment paper and set them aside.

* In the tub of a stand mixer, cream together the butter and brown sugar. Mix for several minutes on medium-high speed with the paddle attachment, until fluffy and light. Just three and a half cups of flour should be used, and the mixture should be blended on low to medium speed.

* Spread half a cup of flour on a large board to avoid the dough from sticking to the top. With a rubber spatula, move the dough to the surface. Knead the dough for five minutes by hand, adding just enough of the additional half cup flour to make a smooth dough. Instead of being oily, the dough should be smooth and pliable, like playdough.

* Split the dough into quarters, wrap securely in plastic wrap, and chill for at least 30 minutes, or until solid enough just to roll out and cut shapes. One-third of the dough should be stretched out to around a 1/2-inch diameter. Using a cookie cutter, sliced into three-by-one rectangular strips, triangles, or shapes. Place each cookie 2 inches apart on a baking sheet. If you're not using sprinkles, make a pattern by poking holes in the cookies with a fork.

* Bake for 15 to 20 minutes, or until golden brown around the edges. If the forms are smaller, bake for less time. To keep the dough chilled and workable, bake it longer for larger shapes, then repeat with the residual dough in batches.

* Allow to cool absolutely on a wire rack before serving. Cookies last a long time when kept at room temperature and sealed airtight.

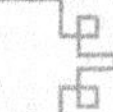

6.6 Macaroons

Preparation time 25 minutes | Servings 24 cookies |
Nutritional facts 75 calories

Ingredients

* 1/2 cup granulated sugar

* 3 cups sweetened shredded coconut

* 4 egg whites

Instructions

The specific rules for making this wonderful meal for women over 50 can be found below. These directives must be followed in the order specified.

* Preheat oven to 350 degrees Fahrenheit.

* After that, cover two sheet pans with parchment paper.

* In a mixing cup, whisk the egg whites until frothy.

* After that, add the sugar and stir well.

* Next, add the coconut and stir with a spoon.

* Next, shovel mounds of cookie dough onto the cookie sheet with a tiny ice cream scoop.

* Bake it for 15 to 20 minutes, or until the surface is golden brown.

* Allow for cooling before feeding.

* Take a bite and rest.

6.7 Goats' Cheese Crostini with Spring Onion & Radish

Preparation time 10 minutes | Servings 7 persons |
Nutritional facts 240 calories

Ingredients

* 10 French breakfast radishes, sliced

* 10 slices of French stick or Ciabatta

* 4,4 oz soft goats' cheese

* 4 spring onions, sliced

* Drizzle of olive oil

Instructions

The specific rules for making this wonderful meal for women over 50 can be found below. These directives must be followed in the order specified.

* Preheat the grill to high.

* Place the bread on a baking sheet after that.

* Drizzle it with olive oil after that.

* Toast each side of the sandwich under the grill until golden brown.

* Spread goats' cheese on each slice after toasting and spread on each slice after toasting. Then garnish with spring onion & radish slices.

* Season it with a pinch of salt and pepper.

* Take a bite and rest.

6.8 Baked Fish and Vegetable Parcels

Preparation time 1 hour 15 minutes | Servings 4persons | Nutritional facts 240 calories

Ingredients

* 2 thinly sliced garlic cloves

* 1 lb of carrots

* 1 lb of courgettes (or 4 medium size)

* A tiny bunch of the parsley, the leaves picked & chopped

* Around 1 cup cider or white wine, tomato passata or vegetable stock

* Black pepper and sea salt

* Bunch of trimmed spring onions

* Cod

* Four fillets of fish (5-7 ozeach)

* Some sprigs of the thyme

* Three to four tbsp. Of olive oil

* Whole grains cooked (1 to 2 oz per serving), for serving

The specific rules for making this wonderful meal for women over 50 can be found below. These directives must be followed in the order specified.

* Preheat the oven to 390 degrees Fahrenheit.

* Have a large baking tray with a rim primed.

* Then, tear off four large sheets of foil or greaseproof paper.

* Cut courgettes into thin ribbons and/or fine slices with a swivel veggie peeler, mandolin, or food processor fitted with a narrow slicing blade. Place the courgettes in a big mixing bowl. Carrots can be sliced in the same manner as courgettes and attached to them.

* In a mixing cup, evenly slice spring onions and blend with thyme, garlic, parsley (if using) and 2 teaspoons olive oil. Season with a pinch of pepper and a pinch of salt to taste. Toss all together well with your mouth.

* Place the vegetables uniformly arranged in the middle of each sheet of paper. Season each fish fillet with salt and pepper before placing it on top of the piles. Gather the sides of the paper and wrap them around the vegetables and fish. Pour a generous quantity of wine, reserve, cider, or passata into each parcel.

* Crimp the top sides of the parcel together. You can completely seal the box if you use foil; if you use cardboard, you can just scrunch it up until the fish is almost covered. Carefully place the parcels on a baking tray. Bake for 15–20 minutes, or until the fish is done and the vegetables are crisp-tender.

* Bring the parcels to the table to the whole grains so that you can drink up the juices.

6.9 Rye and banana cookies

Preparation time 53 minutes | Servings 24 bite sized cookies | Nutritional facts 240 calories

Ingredients

* ½ tsp baking powder

* 3,5 oz extra virgin olive oil, or coconut oil (melted)

* 3,5 oz roughly chopped nuts or mixed seeds

* 4,3 oz raisins or chopped dried apricots

* 4,3 oz dark rye flour

* 5,3 oz porridge oats

* 1 tsp ground mixed spice

* 2 ripe medium bananas, mashed

* 2 tsp ground flaxseed

* 2,6 oz brown sugar

Instructions

The detailed instructions for making this wonderful meal for women over 50 can be found below. These directives must be followed in the order specified.

* Preheat the oven to 350 degrees Fahrenheit.

* First, cover two baking sheets with parchment paper.

* Combine the flour, sugar, oats, baking powder, cinnamon, and ground flaxseed in a big mixing cup. Mix in the dried berries, nuts, and seeds until well mixed, breaking up any stuck-together fruit. Mix in the mashed bananas and the oil until it is well combined.

* Use your fingertips, mould tablespoonfuls of the mixture into thick, circular cookies on the prepared baking sheets. Bake for 12 to 15 minutes, or until the bottoms are golden brown.

* Cool slowly before shifting to a cooling stand to cool fully.

* It can be contained for up to five days in an airtight tin.

6.10 Turkey Meatballs in Tomato Sauce

Preparation time 1 hour 10 minutes | Servings 6 persons |
Nutritional facts 240 calories

Ingredients

*   ½–one tsp of caster sugar (optional)

*   1 beaten egg

*   1 big handful basil leaves

*   1 tsp of fine salt

*   2x1 lb tins tomatoes chopped

*   2 crushed garlic cloves

*   2 crushed or evenly grated garlic cloves

*   2 heaped tbsp. of tomato purée

*   2 small finely diced onion

*   2 tbsp of olive oil

*   2 tsp fresh oregano finely chopped, or one tsp oregano, dried

*   2 tsp hot or mild paprika

*   2 oz Parmesan or pecorino cheese

*   1 lb turkey thighs, minced

*   2 oz white breadcrumbs, fresh

*   2,5 fl oz of whole milk

*   about ¼ freshly grated nutmeg

* black pepper, freshly ground

* salt & pepper

* zest of one lemon finely grated

INSTRUCTIONS

The detailed instructions for making this wonderful meal for women over 50 can be found below. These directives must be followed in the order specified.

* Start by preparing the tomato sauce.

* Take the oil and heat it in a large sauté pan over medium heat.

* Put the onion and a pinch of salt, and fry, stirring periodically, for 5 to 10 minutes, or until softened. After adding the garlic, cook for next 2 minutes.

* Cook for next 2 minutes after adding the paprika & tomato purée.

* Cook for 20 minutes on low heat with the tomatoes and basil. Season with salt, pepper, and a touch of sugar, if necessary, to even out the acidity of the tomatoes.

* In the meantime, make meatballs. In a large mixing cup, spill the milk over the breadcrumbs.

* In a big mixing cup, combine the egg, nutmeg, turkey, oregano, garlic, lemon zest, cinnamon, cheese, and freshly ground black pepper. Blend gently with your paws, taking care not to over-mix. With wet hands, shape the mixture into about twenty small or medium meatballs.

* Carefully put the meatballs in the simmering sauce, cover, and cook for 20 minutes, turning them every ten minutes and shaking the pan periodically.

* Take the cover and cook for an extra 5 minutes. Serve meatballs with basil leaves and gratings of Parmesan or Pecorino cheese.

6.11 Fish pie recipe with pecan crumble

Preparation time 12-15 minutes | Servings 5 persons |
Nutritional facts 240 calories

Ingredients

* 1 small finely chopped dried red chili

* 1 tbsp olive oil, extra virgin

* 1 cup butter beans, washed and rinsed

* 1 oz pecans

* 3 tbsp flat-leaf fresh parsley coarsely chopped, plus more to serve

* 1 oz ground almonds

* 1 oz rolled oats

* 1 oz unsalted butter, cooled & diced

* 4 finely chopped garlic cloves, and also peeled

* 1,4 lb salmon fillets, skinless, cut into 1,2 to 1,6 in pieces

* black pepper freshly ground and Sea salt

* 2 fennel bulbs, the green shoots & tough external sheath discarded, chopped

* 2 x 1 lb tins tomatoes chopped

The specific rules for making this wonderful meal for women over 50 can be found below. These directives must be followed in the order specified.

* Heat the olive oil in an average saucepan over medium heat and add the chilli and garlic. Roast for a few minutes, until the fennel is transparent and slightly softened.

* Reduce to low heat and simmer for 25 to 30 mins, stirring occasionally, until the sauce has thickened, adding parsley, tomatoes, and a pinch of salt and pepper if needed.

* Season the salmon with salt and pepper and sear it in a large non-stick fry pan over high heat, 12 at a time, to gently stain both sides. Gently fold the salmon and butter beans into the sauce, discarding any liquid produced by the fish, and transfer to an ovenproof dish measuring 8x12 in. Filling can be made ahead of time and kept for up to two hours in an airtight bag.

* Whizz pecans until finely minced in a food processor, then add ground almonds, peas, butter, and a pinch of salt and whizz quickly until crumbs hold together in the nibs. This could also be made ahead of time and refrigerated.

* Preheat the oven to 210 degrees Fahrenheit. Sprinkle crumble over pie crust and bake for 30 minutes, or until crumble is finely golden. Serve with a garnish of fresh parsley.

6.12 Spiced carrot & lentil soup

Preparation time 25 minutes | Servings 4 persons |
Nutritional facts 238 calories

Ingredients

* ½ cup of milk

* 5,2 oz split lentils (red)

* 4,2 cups of warm vegetable stock

* 2 tsp of cumin seeds

* 1,3 lb carrots washed & coarsely grated

* A pinch of chili flakes

* Naan bread and plain yogurt, to serve

* Two tbsp of olive oil

Instructions

The specific rules for preparing this delicious meal for women over 50 can be found below. These instructions must be followed in the order specified.

* In a large saucepan, fry 2 teaspoon of cumin seeds and a dash of chili flakes for 1 minute.

* Scoop off about half and set it aside with a spoon. In a saucepan, put 2 tablespoons olive oil, 1,3 lb carrots (coarsely grated), 5,2 oz split red lentils, 4,2 cups hot vegetable stock with ½ cup milk to a boil.

* Cook until the lentils are softened and bloated, around 15 minutes.

* Puree the soup with a stick blender or a food processor until smooth.

* Season to taste, then serve with a dollop of plain yoghurt and a sprinkle of toasted spices on top.

* It is best eaten with warm naan bread.

6.13 Thai prawns with pineapple & green beans

Preparation time 25 minutes | Servings 2 persons |
Nutritional facts 228 calories

Ingredients

* 1 tbsp fish sauce

* 1 tbsp soft brown sugar

* 1 tbsp oil (vegetable)

* 3,5 oz fresh pineapple chunks

* 3,5 oz green bean

* 3,5 oz whole cherry tomato

* 2 lemongrass stalks,

* 2 tbsp liquid chicken stock

* 7 oz raw king prawn

* 4 tbsp lime juice

* small pack basil leaves, regular or Thai

* thumb-sized piece ginger, shredded

INSTRUCTIONS

The specific rules for preparing this delicious meal for women over 50 can be found below. These instructions must be followed in the order specified.

* Mix the sauce ingredients in a shallow dish. After that, put it aside.

* Heat the oil in a broad wok.

* Sauté the ginger and lemongrass until golden brown.

* Stir-fry for 3-5 minutes, or until the beans, pineapple, and cherry tomatoes are only tender. In a mixing dish.

* Combine the sauce and the prawns.

* Stir-fry for another 3 minutes, or cook the prawns. Then, in batches, apply the basil leaves. Lime wedges and basil leaves from the leftovers can be sprinkled on top.

6.14 Paillard of Chicken with Lemon & Herbs

Preparation time 25 minutes | Servings 6 persons |
Nutritional facts 240 calories

INGREDIENTS

We have listed below the ingredients that would be required by you for cooking this healthy and tasty meal meant especially for women observing intermittent fasting:

* 1/2 tbsp balsamic vinegar

* 5,2 oz bag rocket

* 2 garlic cloves

* 2 tbsp olive oil

* 1 oz parmesan

* 3 rosemary sprigs, chopped

* 3 tbsp olive oil

* 6 sage leaves, shredded

* 6 skinless chicken breasts

* Lemon wedges

* Zest 1 lemon and juice of ½

INSTRUCTIONS

The detailed instructions for preparing this delicious meal for women over 50 can be found below. These instructions must be followed in the order specified.

* Sandwich each chicken breast in 2 pieces of baking paper. Using a rolling pin to flatten each chicken piece into 0,2 in thick layer.

* In a serving dish, combine all of the ingredients.

* For marinade, grind the garlic with some salt in a pestle & mortar.

* Combine the sage & rosemary in a beating tub.

* In a mixing bowl, blend the olive oil, lemon juice and zest, and freshly ground black pepper. The marinade should then be poured over the chicken to ensure that it is fully coated. After covering, refrigerate for at least two hours.

* Preheat the grill. The coals should then be spread out evenly until the fires have died out. Cook the chicken about one to two minutes each side. Switch to a board and set aside to cool for a few minutes.

* Add the oil with balsamic vinegar in a bowl and mix. Attach the rocket and season with salt and pepper.

* Serve the salad with the chicken and a squeeze of lemon.

6.15 Chickpea, tomato & spinach curry

Preparation time 45 minutes | Servings 6 persons |
Nutritional facts 204 calories

Ingredients

* ½ tbsp of oil

* 1 chopped onion

* 1 head of broccoli, broken into small florets

* 1 lemon, halved

* 1 tbsp chopped cashews, to mix with the sesame seeds

* 1 tbsp toasted sesame seeds

* 1 tsp of ground cumin

* 1 tsp of turmeric

* 1 tsp of yeast extract (we also used the Marmite)

* 3,5 oz bag baby spinach leaves

* 2 chopped garlic cloves

* 2 tsp of ground coriander

* 1,2 in grated piece of ginger

* 4 tbsp of red lentils

* 1 lb can chickpeas, drained

* 6 tomatoes (ripe)

* 6 tbsp of coconut cream

* pinch of chili flakes

The detailed instructions for preparing this delicious meal for women over 50 can be found below. These instructions must be followed in the order specified.

* To produce a purée, combine the garlic, onion, ginger, and tomatoes in a food processor.

* Next, heat the oil in a wide pan.

* After that, add the spices. After that, fry for a few seconds. Then puree the yeast extract. Mix for two more minutes.

* After that, add the lentils and coconut milk. Cook until the lentils are soft.

* Cook for another four minutes after adding the broccoli.

* Add chickpeas and spinach to the mix. After that, squeeze over the lemon and combine with the sesame and cashews to create a mixture.

* If desired, it can be eaten with brown rice.

6.16 Spiced chicken & pineapple salad

Preparation time 10 minutes | Servings 2 persons |
Nutritional facts 176 calories

INGREDIENTS

* 7,2 oz canned pineapple juice

* 3,4 oz mixed leaf bag

* a handful of halved cherry tomatoes

* about 5,2 oz pack cooked, cut chicken breast (sweet chili, hot & spice, or BBQ)

* 1 red chili, deseeded & chopped

* 1 tbsp sweet chili sauce

* 1 tiny red onion, thinly sliced and halved

* tiny leaves picked bunch coriander

* 2 tbsp vinegar of white wine

INSTRUCTIONS

* Set aside the pineapple juice that has been drained. If the rings are in rings, cut them into chunks.

* Combine the leaves, onion, coriander, chicken, and tomatoes in a mixing bowl and split into two containers if serving as a snack.

* To make the dressing, whisk together 2 tablespoons vinegar, red chilli, pineapple juice, and sweet chilli sauce in a small jam jar or lidded cup with some seasoning, then toss through the salad before serving.

6.17 Broccoli and kale green soup

Preparation time 35 minutes | Servings 2 persons |
Nutritional facts 182 calories

Ingredients

2,1 cups of stock, prepared by mixing one tbsp. of bouillon powder &
boiling water into jug

* 1 lime, zested & juiced

* 1 tbsp of sunflower oil

* 3,5 oz chopped kale

* 2 sliced garlic cloves

* 7 oz roughly sliced courgettes

* 1,2 in/ one in piece turmeric root (fresh)

* 2,8 oz broccoli

* a pinch of Himalayan pink salt

* a small pack of roughly chopped parsley

* half tsp of ground coriander or 1/2 tsp
  of ground turmeric

* thumb-size piece of sliced ginger

INSTRUCTIONS

* Heat the oil in a deep skillet, then add the coriander, garlic, ginger, turmeric, and salt.

* Cook for 2 minutes on moderate flame, then apply three tablespoons of water to moisten the spices.

* Cook for another 3 minutes while adding the courgettes, ensuring that the slices are completely covered with all of the spices. After adding 2,1 cups stock, simmer for three minutes.

* If you are looking for a Add the kale, broccoli, and lime juice to the remaining stock.

* Cook for another 3 to 5 minutes, or until the vegetables are fully tender.

* Turn off the heat and add the chopped parsley to the pan. In a high-powered blender, combine all ingredients and blend until smooth.

* It'll be a pretty green with dark flecks strewn around. Lime zest and parsley may be added as garnishes.

6.18 TERIYAKI SALMON PARCELS

Preparation time 35 minutes | Servings 4 persons |
Nutritional facts 243 calories

INGREDIENTS

* 1 tbsp of clear honey

* 1 tbsp of mirin (optional)

* 2 tbsp soy sauce, low salt

* 10,5 oz tender stem broccoli

* 4 x 3,5 oz salmon fillets

* Little bit of sunflower oil

* One finely chopped garlic clove

* One small ginger piece, cut into matchsticks

* Sesame oil, a little (optional)

* Spring onions (sliced)

* Sesame seeds (toasted)

INSTRUCTIONS

* Prepare both the sauce and the marinade.

* Mix the soy sauce, garlic, butter, and mirin in a small bowl and set aside. The foil squares can be removed. Using scissors, cut four squares of foil measuring roughly 11,8 in.

* To bring the sides up a bit, rub a little oil onto each sheet of foil.

* Fill the parcels to the brim. Place a few broccoli stems on top of each, followed by the salmon fillet and ginger.

* Drizzle the sauce over the top. Pour the sauce over each salmon fillet and drizzle with sesame oil if needed.

* Place the packages in a sealed envelope. Fold the foil edges together and position them on a baking sheet to secure the packets. It's possible to plan ahead of time up to a day.

* Prepare the parcels. Preheat the oven to 180-200 °F fan/gas 6

* After that, bake the parcels for 15 to 20 minutes.

* Set aside for a few more minutes after that. Place each parcel on a plate and give each individual the opportunity to open it. Serve with rice and a sprinkling of spring onions and sesame seeds on the side

6.19 Turkish One-Pan Eggs & Peppers

Preparation time 25 minutes | Servings 2 persons |
Nutritional facts 240 calories

Ingredients

* 1 red or green pepper

* 1-2 red chili

* 1-2 tsp caster sugar

* 2 garlic cloves, crushed

* 2 onions, sliced

* 2 tbsp olive oil

* 4 eggs

* 1 lb can chopped tomatoes

* 6 tbsp thick, creamy yogurt

* small bunch parsley, roughly chopped

Instructions

* Heat the oil in a frying pan. In a mixing dish, combine the onions, pepper, and chilies.

* Cook until they begin to soften. Combine the tomatoes and sugar in a large mixing bowl. Season with salt and pepper until the liquid has been reduced.

* Using a wooden spoon, make four pockets in the tomato mixture and crack the eggs into them.

* Cook the eggs, sealed, on low heat until they are only set. After combining the yoghurt with the garlic, season with salt and pepper.

* Serve immediately with parsley and a dollop of garlic-flavoured yoghurt straight from the pan.

6.20 Asian chicken salad

Preparation time 20 minutes | Servings 2 persons |
Nutritional facts 109 calories

INGREDIENTS

* ¼ sliced cucumber lengthways halved

* ¼ thinly sliced red onion

* ½ chili, seeds removed & thinly cut

* ½ lime zest & juice (around 1 tbsp)

* 1 chicken breast boneless & skinless

* 1 tbsp of fish sauce

* 1 tsp of caster sugar

* 3,5 oz salad leaves bag mixed

* big handful of roughly chopped coriander

INSTRUCTIONS

* Put the chicken in a cold-water tank. Then bring to the boil and reduce to a low heat for 10 minutes. Remove the meat from pan and slice it with a fork.

* Stir together the lime zest, fish sauce, milk, and sugar until the sugar is fully dissolved.

*   Mix the leaves and coriander in a container.

Then add the chicken, chili, cucumber, and cabbage to the top. Place the dressing in a separate dish.

Extra content (pdf to print)

Write to us to receive your extra content…

… Food diary as a gift!!!

To receive your gift click below.

https://forms.gle/AUoUHahY565G5GF18

Thanks for reading this far!

I would be grateful if you could take a minute of your time to leave an honest Amazon review about my work, so that we can share your experience with other customers.

Thanks again!

CONCLUSION

Even if you adjust the timing of when you eat foods, it is still best to check with a competent medical professional before making dietary adjustments. They will help you figure out if intermittent fasting is right for you. It is particularly important for longer-term fasts, which can lead to vitamin and mineral depletion. Its critical to recognize that our bodies are extremely intelligent. If food is limited at one meal, the body can experience increased hunger and calorie consumption at the next meal and a slowing of metabolism to match calorie consumption. While intermittent fasting has many potential health benefits, it should not be assumed that it would result in massive weight loss and delay the diseases spread or progression if strictly observed.

It's a valuable tool, but in this case, a combination of tools would be needed to achieve and sustain optimal health. Intermittent fasting is a diet that includes periods of fasting and encourages the body to burn fat. During the fasting period (usually 16 hours), the body undergoes changes that promote enhanced longevity, tissue regeneration, reduced inflammation, and body weight hormonal regulation changes.

Intermittent fasting is a relatively simple diet to adapt to and can be an effective diet for many people, but it is not suitable for someone who is insulin-dependent or needs regularly timed meals. So, Intermittent fasting is the best way to control your health at an advanced age when your body is constantly changing, even with the slightest change in your diet plan.

> # Will is power,
> ## the rest is just exuses!!!